Table of Contents

Cannabidiol (CBD) oil is a naturally oc¬curring constituent of industrial hemp and marijuana, which are collectively called cannabis. CBD oil is 1 of at least 85 can¬nabinoid compounds found in cannabis and is popular for its medicinal benefits. After tetrahydrocannabinol (THC), CBD oil is the second-most-abundant compo¬nent of cannabis. Other names for CBD oil include CBD-rich hemp oil, hemp-derived CBD oil, or CBD-rich cannabis oil. Con-sidered to be generally safe, CBD has been used medicinally for decades. However, CBD is not medical marijuana and should be distinguished from high-CBD strains of medical marijuana, which do contain THC, such as "Charlotte's Web."

The most abundant compound in can¬nabis, THC is also a cannabinoid. The THC component induces the psychoac¬tive effect, "high." A cannabis plant has different amounts of CBD and THC depending on the strain and thus provides different recreational or medicinal effects. The cannabinoid profile of industrial hemp or medical marijuana is ideal for people looking for the medical benefits of CBD without the "high" of the THC.

The mechanism of action of CBD is multifold.[1-3] Two cannabinoid receptors are known to exist in the human body: CB1 and CB2 receptors. The CB1 recep¬tors are located mainly in the brain and modulate neurotransmitter release in a manner that prevents excessive neuronal activity (thus calming and decreasing anxiety), as well as reduces pain, reduces inflammation, regulates movement and posture control, and regulates sensory perception, memory, and cognitive func¬tion. An endogenous ligand, anandamide, which occurs naturally in our bodies, binds to the CB1 receptors through the G-protein coupling system. CBD has an indirect effect on the CB1 receptors by stopping the enzymatic breakdown of anandamide, allowing it to stay in the sys¬tem longer and provide medical benefits. CBD has a mild effect on the CB2 recep¬tors, which are located in the periphery in lymphoid tissue. CBD helps to mediate the release of cytokines from the immune cells in a manner that helps to reduce inflam¬mation and pain.

Other mechanisms of action of CBD include stimulation of vanilloid pain recep¬tors (TRPV-1 receptor), which are known to mediate pain perception, inflamma¬tion, and body temperature. In addition, CBD may exert its anti-anxiety effect by activating adenosine receptors which play a significant role in cardiovascular function and cause a broad anti-inflammatory effect throughout the body. At high concentra¬tions, CBD directly activates the 5-HT1A serotonin receptor, thereby conferring an antidepressant effect. Cannabidiol has been found to be an antagonist at the po-tentially new third cannabinoid receptor, GPR55, in the caudate nucleus and puta¬men, which if stimulated may contribute to osteoporosis.

Since the 1940s, a considerable number of published articles have dealt with the chemistry, biochemistry, pharmacology, and clinical effects of CBD. The last de¬cade has shown a notable increase in the scientific literature on CBD, owing to its identification for reducing nausea and vomiting, combating psychotic disorders, reducing inflammation, decreasing anxi¬ety and depression, improving sleep, and increasing a sense of well-being. Find¬ings presented at the 2015 International Cannabinoid Research Society at its 25th Annual Symposium reported the use of CBD as beneficial for kidney fibrosis and inflammation, metabolic syndrome, over¬weight and obesity, anorexia-cachexia syn¬drome, and modification of osteoarthritic and other musculoskeletal conditions.

Although studies have demonstrated the calming, anti-inflammatory, and relaxing effects of CBD, clinical data from actual cases is minimal. This case study offers evidence that CBD is effective as a safe alternative treatment to traditional psy-chiatric medications for reducing anxiety and insomnia.

Fear and anxiety are adaptive responses essential to coping with threats to survival. Yet excessive or persistent fear may be maladaptive, leading to disability. Symptoms arising from excessive fear and anxiety occur in a number of neuropsychiatric disorders, including generalized anxiety disorder (GAD), panic disorder (PD), post-traumatic stress disorder (PTSD), social anxiety disorder (SAD), and obsessive–compulsive disorder (OCD). Notably, PTSD and OCD are no longer classified as anxiety disorders in the recent revision of the Diagnostic and Statistical Manual of Mental Disorders; however, excessive anxiety is central to the symptomatology of both disorders.

These anxiety-related disorders are associated with a diminished sense of well-being, elevated rates of unemployment and relationship breakdown, and elevated suicide risk. Together, they have a lifetime prevalence in the USA of 29 %, the highest of any mental disorder, and constitute an immense social and economic burden.

Currently available pharmacological treatments include serotonin reuptake inhibitors, serotonin–norepinephrine reuptake inhibitors, benzodiazepines, monoamine oxidase inhibitors, tricyclic antidepressant drugs, and partial 5-

hydroxytryptamine (5-HT)1A receptor agonists. Anticonvulsants and atypical antipsychotics are also used to treat PTSD. These medications are associated with limited response rates and residual symptoms, particularly in PTSD, and adverse effects may also limit tolerability and adherence. The substantial burden of anxiety-related disorders and the limitations of current treatments place a high priority on developing novel pharmaceutical treatments.

Cannabidiol (CBD) is a phytocannabinoid constituent of Cannabis sativa that lacks the psychoactive effects of tetrahydrocannabinol (THC). CBD has broad therapeutic properties across a range of neuropsychiatric disorders, stemming from diverse central nervous system actions. In recent years, CBD has attracted increasing interest as a potential anxiolytic treatment. The purpose of this review is to assess evidence from current preclinical, clinical, and epidemiological studies pertaining to the potential risks and benefits of CBD as a treatment for anxiety disorders.

CBD PHARMACOLOGY RELEVANT TO ANXIETY

General Pharmacology and Therapeutic Profile Cannabis sativa, a species of the Cannabis genus of flowering plants, is one of the most frequently used illicit recreational substances in Western culture. The 2 major phyto-cannabinoid constituents with central nervous system activity are THC, responsible for the euphoric and mind-altering effects, and CBD, which lacks these psychoactive effects. Preclinical and clinical studies show CBD possesses a wide range of therapeutic properties, including antipsychotic, analgesic, neuroprotective, anticonvulsant, antiemetic, antioxidant, anti-inflammatory, antiarthritic, and antineoplastic properties. A review of potential side effects in humans found that CBD was well tolerated across a wide dose range, up to 1500 mg/day (orally), with no reported psychomotor slowing, negative mood effects, or vital sign abnormalities noted.

CBD has a broad pharmacological profile, including interactions with several receptors known to regulate fear and anxiety-related behaviors, specifically the cannabinoid type 1 receptor (CB1R), the serotonin 5-HT1A receptor, and the transient receptor potential (TRP) vanilloid type 1 (TRPV1) receptor. In addition, CBD may also regulate, directly or indirectly, the peroxisome proliferator-activated receptor-γ, the orphan G-protein-coupled receptor 55, the equilibrative nucleoside transporter, the adenosine transporter, additional TRP channels, and glycine receptors. In the current review of primary studies, the following receptor-specific actions were found to have been investigated as potential mediators of CBD's anxiolytic action: CB1R, TRPV1 receptors, and 5-HT1A receptors. Pharmacology relevant to these actions is detailed below.

THE ENDOCANNABINOID SYSTEM

Following cloning of the endogenous receptor for THC, namely the CB1R, endogenous CB1R ligands, or

Bendocannabinoids (ECBs) were discovered, namely anandamide (AEA) and 2-arachidonoylglycerol.

The CB1R is an inhibitory Gi/o protein-coupled receptor that is mainly localized to nerve terminals, and is expressed on both γ-aminobutryic acid-ergic and glutamatergic neurons. ECBs are fatty acid derivatives that are synthesized on demand in response to neuronal depolarization and Ca2+ influx, via cleavage of membrane phospholipids. The primary mechanism by which ECBs regulate synaptic function is retrograde signaling, wherein ECBs produced by depolarization of the postsynaptic neuron activate presynaptic CB1Rs, leading to inhibition of neurotransmitter release. The BECB system includes AEA and 2-arachidonoylglycerol; their respective degradative enzymes fatty acid amide hydroxylase (FAAH) and monoacylglycerol lipase; the CB1R and related CB2 receptor (the latter expressed mainly in the periphery); as well as several other receptors activated by ECBs, including the TRPV1 receptor, peroxisome proliferator-activated receptor-γ, and G protein-coupled 55 receptor, which functionally interact with CB1R signaling.

Interactions with the TRPV1 receptor, in particular, appear to be critical in regulating the extent to which ECB release leads to inhibition or facilitation of presynaptic neurotransmitter release. The TRPV1 receptor is a postsynaptic cation channel that underlies sensation of noxious heat in the periphery, with capsacin (hot chili) as an exogenous ligand. TRPV1 receptors are also expressed in the brain, including the amygdala, periaqueductal grey, hippocampus, and other areas.

The ECB system regulates diverse physiological functions, including caloric energy balance and immune function.

The ECB system is also integral to regulation of emotional behavior, being essential to forms of synaptic plasticity that determine learning and response to emotionally salient, particularly highly aversive events. Activation of CB1Rs produces anxiolytic effects in various models of unconditioned fear, relevant to multiple anxiety disorder symptom domains. Regarding conditioned fear, the effect of CB1R activation is complex: CB1R activation may enhance or reduce fear expression, depending on brain locus and the ECB ligand; however, CB1R activation potently enhances fear extinction, and can prevent fear reconsolidation. Genetic manipulations that impede CB1R activation are anxiogenic, and individuals with ECB system gene polymorphisms that reduce ECB tone—for example, FAAH gene polymorphisms—exhibit physiological, psychological, and neuroimaging features consistent with impaired fear regulation. Reduction of AEA–CB1R signaling in the amygdala mediates the anxiogenic effects of corticotropin-releasing hormone, and CB1R activation is essential to negative feedback of the neuroendocrine stress response, and protects against the adverse effects of chronic stress. Finally, chronic stress impairs ECB signaling in the hippocampus and amygdala, leading to anxiety, and people with PTSD show elevated CB1R availability and reduced peripheral AEA, suggestive of reduced ECB tone. Accordingly, CB1R activation has been suggested as a target for anxiolytic drug development. Proposed agents for enhancing CB1R activation include THC, which is a potent and direct agonist; synthetic CB1R agonists; FAAH inhibitors and other agents that increase ECB availability, as well as nonpsychoactive cannabis phytocannabinoids, including CBD. While CBD has low affinity for the CB1R, it functions as an indirect agonist, potentially via augmentation of CB1R constitutional activity, or via increasing AEA through FAAH inhibition.

Several complexities of the ECB system may impact upon the potential of CBD and other CB1R-activating agents to serve as anxiolytic drugs. First, CB1R agonists, including THC and AEA, have a biphasic effect: low doses are anxiolytic, but higher doses are ineffective or anxiogenic, in both preclinical models in and humans. This biphasic profile may stem from the capacity of CB1R agonists to also activate TRPV1 receptors when administered at a high, but not low dose, as demonstrated for AEA. Activation of TRPV1 receptors is predominantly anxiogenic, and thus a critical balance of ECB levels, determining CB1 versus TRPV1 Activation, is proposed to govern emotional behavior.

CBD acts as a TRPV1 agonist at high concentrations, potentially by interfering with AEA inactivation. In addition to dose-dependent activation of TRPV1 channels, the anxiogenic versus anxiolytic balance of CB1R agonists also depends on dynamic factors, including environmental stressors.

5-HT1A RECEPTORS

The 5-HT1A receptor (5-HT1AR) is an established anxiolytic target. Buspirone and other 5-HT1AR agonists are approved for the treatment of GAD, with fair response rates. In preclinical studies, 5-HT1AR agonists are anxiolytic in animal models of general anxiety, prevent the adverse effects of stress, and enhance fear extinction. Both pre- and postsynaptic 5-HT1ARs are coupled to various members of the Gi/o protein family. They are expressed on serotonergic neurons in the raphe, where they exert autoinhibitory function, and various other brain areas involved in fear and anxiety. Mechanisms underlying the anxiolytic effects of 5-HT1AR activation are complex, varying between both brain region, and pre- versus postsynaptic locus, and are not fully established. While in vitro studies suggest CBD acts as a direct 5-HT1AR agonist, in vivo studies are more consistent with CBD acting as an allosteric modulator, or facilitator of 5-HT1A signaling.

Generalized Anxiety Models

CBD has been studied in a wide range of animal models of general anxiety, including the elevated plus maze (EPM), the Vogel-conflict test (VCT), and the elevated T maze (ETM). Initial studies of CBD in these models showed conflicting results: high (100 mg/kg) doses were ineffective, while low (10 mg/kg) doses were anxiolytic. When tested over a wide range of doses in further studies, the anxiolytic effects of CBD presented a bell-shaped dose–response curve, with anxiolytic effects observed at moderate but not higher doses. All further studies of acute systemic CBD without prior stress showed anxiolytic effects or no effect, the latter study involving intracerebroventricular rather than the intraperitoneal route. No anxiogenic effects of acute systemic CBD dosing in models of general anxiety have yet been reported. As yet, few studies have examined chronic dosing effects of CBD in models of generalized anxiety.

Campos et al. showed that in rat, CBD treatment for 21 days attenuated inhibitory avoidance acquisition.

Long et al. showed that, in mouse, CBD produced moderate anxiolytic effects in some paradigms, with no effects in others.

Anxiolytic effects of CBD in models of generalized anxiety have been linked to specific receptor mechanisms and brain regions. The midbrain dorsal periaqueductal gray (DPAG) is integral to anxiety, orchestrating autonomic and behavioral responses to threat, and DPAG stimulation in humans produces feelings of intense distress and dread. Microinjection of CBD into the DPAG produced anxiolytic effects in the EPM, VGC, and ETM that were partially mediated by activation of 5-HT1ARs but not by CB1Rs. The bed nucleus of the stria terminalis (BNST) serves as a principal output structure of the amygdaloid complex to coordinate sustained fear responses, relevant to anxiety. Anxiolytic effects of CBD in the

EPM and VCT occurred upon microinjection into the BNST, where they depended on 5-HT1AR activation, and also upon microinjection into the central nucleus of the amygdala. In the prelimbic cortex, which drives expression of fear responses via connections with the amygdala, CBD had more complex effects: in unstressed rats, CBD was anxiogenic in the EPM, partially via 5-HT1AR receptor activation; however, following acute restraint stress, CBD was anxiolytic.

Finally, the anxiolytic effects of systemic CBD partially depended on GABAA receptor activation in the EPM model but not in the VCT model.

As noted, CBD has been found to have a bell-shaped response curve, with higher doses being ineffective. This may reflect activation of TRPV1 receptors at higher dose, as blockade of TRPV1 receptors in the DPAG rendered a previously ineffective high dose of CBD as anxiolytic in the EPM. Given TRPV1 receptors have anxiogenic effects, this may indicate that at higher doses, CBD's interaction with TRPV1 receptors to some extent impedes anxiolytic actions, although was notably not sufficient to produce anxiogenic effects.

Stress is an important contributor to anxiety disorders, and traumatic stress exposure is essential to the development of PTSD. Systemically administered CBD reduced acute increases in heart rate and blood pressure induced by restraint stress, as well as the delayed (24h) anxiogenic effects of stress in the EPM, partially by 5-HT1AR activation. However intra-BNST microinjection of CBD augmented stress-induced heart rate increase, also partially via 5-HT1AR activation. In a subchronic study, CBD administered daily 1h after predator stress (a proposed model of PTSD) reduced the long-lasting anxiogenic effects of chronic predator stress, partially via 5-HT1AR activation. In a chronic study, systemic CBD prevented increased anxiety produced by chronic unpredictable stress, in addition to increasing hippocampal AEA; these anxiolytic effects depended upon CB1R activation and hippocampal neurogenesis, as demonstrated by genetic ablation techniques. Prior stress also appears to modulate CBD's anxiogenic effects: microinjection of CBD into the prelimbic cortex of unstressed animals was anxiogenic in the EPM but following restraint stress was found to be anxiolytic. Likewise, systemic CBD was anxiolytic in the EPM following but not prior to stress.

PD AND COMPULSIVE BEHAVIOR MODELS

CBD inhibited escape responses in the ETM and increased DPAG escape electrical threshold, both proposed models of panic attacks. These effects partially depended on 5-HT1AR activation but were not affected by CB1R blockade. CBD was also panicolytic in the predator–prey model, which assesses explosive escape and defensive immobility in response to a boa constrictor snake, also partially via

5-HT1AR activation; however, more consistent with an anxiogenic effect, CBD was also noted to decrease time spent outside the burrow and increase defensive attention.

Finally, CBD, partially via CB1Rs, decreased defensive immobility and explosive escape caused by bicuculline-induced neuronal activation in the superior colliculus. Anticompulsive effects of CBD were investigated in marble-burying behavior, conceptualized to model OCD. Acute systemic CBD reduced marble-burying behavior for up to 7 days, with no attenuation in effect up to high (120 mg/kg) doses, and effect shown to depend on CB1Rs but not 5-HT1ARs. CBD for Anxiety We all get anxious at some point in our lives. However, is this really healthy and do we manage it correctly? Furthermore, just how or when do you know that your anxiety is getting out of hand and what is the best way of treating it?

ANXIETY

Anxiety is a feeling that is often characterized by intense fear, worry, or nervousness, typically about an imminent event or something with an uncertain outcome. It can be distracting at best and all-consuming at worst.

Anxiety is normal in our lives and can actually be desirable because it's a critical adaptive response that helps us avoid problems and strive to be safe. That fear that things might go wrong somehow motivates us to stay on track and act more responsibly.

For instance, anxiety can make you work harder to improve your situations like work and relationships. Also, a student that is anxious about their results is bound to study harder just because of that fear of failing. It is also manageable and outbreaks can be prevented through maintaining a healthy lifestyle, for example, a healthy diet, regular exercise and maintaining regular sleep patterns. However, when we don't manage anxiety effectively, consistent long-lasting anxiety can result in the form of an anxiety disorder. This is a beast that needs to be dealt with immediately before it leads to medical and mental illnesses.

In case you're wondering how you would know when your anxiety is getting out of hand, here are a few clues. Anxiety disorder can be characterized by uneasy body reactions some of which include panic attacks, cold or sweat outbreaks, insomnia, nausea, dry mouth, and tense muscles.

There are different types of anxieties which can be grouped in the following ways:

• General anxiety – This is a chronic disorder where you have long-lasting anxiety and worry about non-specific life events.

• Social phobia -This is a type of anxiety where you get scared of different social situations.

• Panic disorder – This is where anxiety and fear arise frequently and without reasonable cause. It is characterized by sudden panic attacks, chest pain, and heart attacks.

- Post-Traumatic stress disorder – This is a type of anxiety that is caused by an unfortunate event happens in your life, leaving a huge negative impact.

- Obsessive-compulsive disorder – This is a type of anxiety that makes you become extremely obsessed with things or even people. The victims also experience constant hallucinations.

Anxiety may be caused by a mental condition, a physical condition, the effects of drugs, or a combination of these. The doctor's initial task is to see if your anxiety is a symptom of another medical condition.

Common causes of anxiety include these mental conditions:

• Panic disorder: In addition to anxiety, common symptoms of panic disorders are palpitations (feeling your heart beat), dizziness, and shortness of breath. These same symptoms also can be caused by coffee (caffeine), amphetamines ("speed" is the street slang for amphetamines when they are not prescribed by a doctor), an overactive thyroid, abnormal heart rhythms, and other heart abnormalities (such as mitral valve prolapse).

- Generalized anxiety disorder

- Phobic disorders

- Stress disorders

These common external factors can cause anxiety:

- Stress at work

- Stress from school

- Stress in a personal relationship such as marriage

- Financial stress

- Stress from an emotional trauma such as the death of a loved one

- Stress from a serious medical illness

- Side effect of medication

- Use of an illicit drug, such as cocaine

- Symptom of a medical illness (such as heart attack, heat stroke, hypoglycemia)

- Lack of oxygen in circumstances as diverse as high altitude sickness, emphysema, or pulmonary embolism (a blood clot in the vessels of the lung).

Having looked at what anxiety is, the various symptoms, and the different types of anxieties, the obvious question now is; how do you treat anxiety disorders?

It is clear that an anxiety disorder is not something anyone could wish to live with. It affects individuals psychologically, physically and emotionally thus generally impacting negatively on their health. Therefore, this gives us more than enough reasons to get the best way of treating it.

There are various methods which people use to treat anxiety, with the most famous one being the use of antidepressants. Frequently treatments consist of a combination of psychotherapy and behavioral therapy. However, at the end of the day, you don't want to keep doing trial and error to treat your anxiety! So what is the surest way of treatment?

Well, research has proven that CBD is a long-term and natural solution to anxiety issues as well as other several health conditions.

What Is CBD?

CBD (Cannabidiol) is one of the active ingredients found in Cannabis, a famous plant that has over 65 active ingredients. CBD, however, is not psychoactive. It is not like some other ingredients that are found in cannabis, for instance, THC (Tetrahydrocannabinol). THC is another active ingredient in Cannabis and is a known psychoactive substance.

Though CBD has significant levels of cannabis sativa, it doesn't cause the psychoactivity that marijuana does. This is what makes it acceptable by the medical community as a genuine treatment option. It's a pharmacologically broad-spectrum drug that has grown increasing interest and has been used in the past few years as a treatment for a range of neuropsychiatric disorders. Consequently, it has been proven to be an effective treatment not only for anxiety but also other related disorders. Other conditions that can be treated by CBD include depression, pain, neurodegenerative disorders (e.g. dementia), blood pressure, lactose intolerance, and epilepsy.

CANNABIS, MOOD, AND DEPRESSION

Cannabis use has commonly been reported not only to reduce anxiety but also to enhance mood and cause euphoria. Indeed, pre-clinical animal data suggest that THC (at lower doses) and CBD both produce anti-depressant effects. This suggests that cannabis use might be effective in reducing depression; however, the reports of cannabis as an anti-depressant are contradictory. Self-report questionnaires examining reasons for cannabis use found that 22 percent of their sample used cannabis to reduce depression. Indeed, a questionnaire on depressive symptoms in a survey of nearly 4500 people revealed fewer depressive symptoms in cannabis users than in non-users. Case reports of five people suffering from depression revealed that depression preceded cannabis use and that the effects of cannabis had some anti-depressant effects. In addition, cannabis use is associated with elevated mood and decreased depression in patients with chronic diseases. On the other hand, oral THC administration to depressed individuals can also result in dysphoria in some patients, especially those who are naïve to the psychoactive effects of cannabis. Furthermore, pure THC has been reported to increase anxiety when given alone, whereas co-administration of CBD can counter its effect. [Without the benefit of the additional cannabinoid compounds (especially CBD) pure THC often does not have the same effect as cannabis consumption.

MARIJUANA FOR "ANXIETY-TENSION"

The possibility that a woman could have painless labor became an idée fixe of H. L. ("Doc") Humes, a literary wunderkind and MIT science prodigy who developed some intriguing theories about cannabis. When his wife was giving birth at their home on July 4, 1977, they tried an experiment involving marijuana, breathing exercises, and massage. Humes gave her some pot to inhale just before each contraction and this helped her immensely.

Marijuana is "among the most forgiving medicines we know," said Humes, who described cannabis as a "neurological laxative" that "acts to surface anxiety which the user holds within himself." Doc touted the weed as the best remedy for stress, "the necessary medicine for the nation's anxiety-tension problem."

"America is so sick," he declared, "and cannabis is the specific medicine for the disease that afflicts us."

Chronic "anxiety-tension," Humes explained, "is a state of general blockage that shows up most obviously at an individual's 'weakest link,' so it can have a wide variety of physical and emotional symptoms, as well as being generally debilitating ... Most of the common elements from which people suffer are really symptoms of anxiety-tension, including headache, backache, insomnia, fatigue, irritability, GI disturbances such as constipation and ulcers, overweight, arthritis, and so on. Anxiety-tension has also been very clearly implicated in more deadly disorders such as high blood pressure, heart disease, cancer proneness, and premature aging … Depression is frequently a symptom of anxiety-tension."

"The medical use of cannabis depends precisely on managing its psychoactive properties. In heavy dosage, it functions like a hypnotic. In a light dosage it functions like an illuminant." — H.L. (Doc) Humes

Ganja's biphasic qualities allow smokers to "equilibriate" the nervous system, according to Humes. Consumed in appropriate quantities, the herb could calm the hyper or invigorate the sluggish. "The medical use of cannabis depends precisely on managing its psychoactive properties," Doc counseled. "In heavy dosage, it functions like a hypnotic. In a light dosage it functions like an illuminant."

Humes saw early on that the widespread "recreational use of cannabis is also a form of self-medication," even if most marijuana smokers did not acknowledge this to themselves. He lamented the fact that hundreds of thousands of young people are arrested each year for using the most efficacious and least harmful medication available to cope with the stress of living in the modern world.

CBD (Cannabidiol) treats anxiety by working on one's serotonin levels through a cannabinoid receptor effect. It directly impacts on the stress responses which are obviously mental.

With CBD oil, you have cannabinoid receptors all over your body, including in your skin and digestive tract. What CBD oil does is it binds to the cannabinoid receptors in your body, thus affecting the endocannabinoid system. This helps with inflammation, mood, memory, immune system, reproduction, pain perception, sleep, and appetite. CBD oil has clearly proven itself as a therapeutic remedy to help a variety of ailments.

There is sufficient evidence from the research that has been done over the recent years that CBD actually treats anxiety by alleviating the fear responses produced in individuals' minds.

Studies done on animals with anxiety as well as on healthy volunteers proved that CBD can be used as an anxiolytic drug. It was also shown to reduce anxiety in patients with social anxiety disorder, one of the most common anxiety conditions that impair a person's social life.

DOSAGE

CBD is still in its early stages of research and thus determining the particular dosage for each individual is a bit tricky. Your current source of CBD oil will also determine its strength and bioavailability. This is because medication prescription is determined by a variety of factors, for instance, weight, age and the strength of the medicine. Putting these factors into consideration, you need to keep these two things in mind:

1. Introduce small doses of CBD for a start.

2. Maintain the same dosage for a few days to assess the results before increasing it.

Commencing slowly and increasing the dose gradually ensures that you're not overdosing or wasting your CBD oil. This enables you to identify the perfect dosage that works for your specific condition instead of relying on information that probably suits a different individual.

Just to guide you more on how to start, scientific research indicates that an amount of 40 mg per day is recommended for beginners.

One might wonder; why use CBD to treat anxiety when you can easily use antidepressants? In most scenarios, people use antidepressants whenever faced with anxiety disorders. The antidepressants only suppress the anxiety but don't actually deal with the root problem. This makes people become hopelessly dependent on them since the moment they stop using them, the anxiety automatically returns even worse than before.

Nevertheless, the side effects are concerning. A long-term use of anti-depressants also puts a heavy strain on the patient's kidney to cleanse the blood from the chemicals contained in them.

Considering that some drugs must be taken daily, anti-depressants are not a good option. They are also extremely addictive and result in withdrawal symptoms when discontinued, for example, dizziness, headache, and nausea. This is where CBD is different. CBD is not a psychoactive substance, so there is no danger of getting "high" from it. There are also no harmful side effects or withdrawal symptoms when using CBD products. This qualifies it to be a risk-free treatment that can also help with other health problems like digestive issues, insomnia, and stress. For your information, the main reason why CBD has gotten so much of the spotlight lately is that CBD oil has helped people with rare conditions such as the Dravet syndrome, a rare form of epilepsy that is hard to treat. People have been enabled to cut down the numerous number of seizures to zero within a week.

HOW IS IT ADMINISTERED?

First things first; before using any type of CBD; you must ensure you are using a high-quality brand. There are a lot of scammers out there. The best way of obtaining the product is by ordering from pharmacies where you need a prescription or through a high-quality brand, for example, Elixinol. However, before going down the CBD oil route, it is always best to consult with your doctor to understand which CBD oil is best for you.

Here are some of the things that you should consider before getting started:

- Do I have an anxiety disorder or simple daily stress?

- Do I need to combine THC with CBD?

- What's my main consideration – price or strength?

- What are the legal restrictions in my state?

Please note that there are two primary ways to supplement with CBD oil to treat anxiety and depression. You can take pure CBD oil that has no THC (e.g. CBD hemp oil), Or you can take CBD oil with THC to get the benefits of both (e.g. Cannabis oil).

SUMMARY AND CLINICAL RELEVANCE

Overall, existing preclinical evidence strongly supports the potential of CBD as a treatment for anxiety disorders. as a treatment for anxiety disorders.

CBD exhibits a broad range of actions, relevant to multiple symptom domains, including anxiolytic, panicolytic, and anticompulsive actions, as well as a decrease in autonomic arousal, a decrease in conditioned fear expression, enhancement of fear extinction, reconsolidation blockade, and prevention of the long-term anxiogenic effects of stress. Activation of 5-HT1ARs appears to mediate anxiolytic and panicolytic effects, in addition to reducing conditioned fear expression, although CB1R activation may play a limited role.

By contrast, CB1R activation appears to mediate CBD's anti- compulsive effects, enhancement of fear extinction, reconsolidation blockade, and capacity to prevent the long-term anxiogenic consequences of stress, with involvement of hippocampal neurogenesis.

While CBD predominantly has acute anxiolytic effects, some species discrepancies are apparent. In addition, effects may be contingent on prior stress and vary according to brain region. A notable contrast between CBD and other agents that target the ECB system, including THC, direct CB1R agonists and FAAH inhibitors, is a lack of anxiogenic effects at a higher dose. Further receptor-specific studies may elucidate the receptor specific basis of this distinct dose response profile.

Further studies are also required to establish the efficacy of CBD when administered in chronic dosing, as relatively few relevant studies exist, with mixed results, including both anxiolytic and anxiogenic outcomes.

Overall, preclinical evidence supports systemic CBD as an acute treatment of GAD, SAD, PD, OCD, and PTSD, and suggests that CBD has the advantage of not producing anxiogenic effects at higher dose, as distinct from other agents that enhance CB1R activation. In particular, results show potential for the treatment of multiple PTSD symptom domains, including reducing arousal and avoidance, preventing the long-term adverse effects of stress, as well as enhancing the extinction and blocking the reconsolidation of persistent fear memories.

Human Experimental and Clinical Studies

Evidence from Acute Psychological Studies.

The anxiolytic effects of CBD in humans were first demonstrated in the context of reversing the anxiogenic effects of

THC. CBD reduced THC-induced anxiety when administered simultaneously with this agent, but had no effect on baseline anxiety when administered alone. Further studies using higher doses supported a lack of anxiolytic effects at baseline.

By contrast, CBD potently reduces experimentally induced anxiety or fear. CBD reduced anxiety associated with a simulated public speaking test in healthy subjects, and in subjects with SAD, showing a comparable efficacy to ipsapirone (a 5- HT1AR agonist) or diazepam. CBD also reduced the presumed anticipatory anxiety associated with undergoing a single-photon emission computed tomography (SPECT) imaging procedure, in both healthy and SAD subjects.

Finally, CBD enhanced extinction of fear memories in healthy volunteers: specifically, inhaled CBD administered prior to or after extinction training in a contextual fear conditioning paradigm led to a trend-level enhancement in the reduction of skin conductance response during reinstatement, and a significant reduction in expectancy (of shock) ratings during reinstatement.

CBD for anxiety is a scientifically proven way of treating anxiety. Animal studies have characterized the details of how CBD acts on the brain, and human studies of patients with and without anxiety disorders have started to validate CBD's efficacy as an anti-anxiety treatment.

With the current huge social and financial costs of anxiety disorders, CBD has the potential to play a significant role in treating a multitude of anxiety-related disorders.